MW00474316

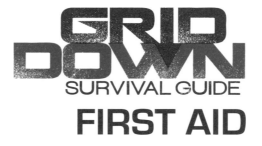

GRID DOWN SURVIVAL GUIDE

FIRST AID

AARON IWANCIW

Grid Down Survival Guide
FIRST AID

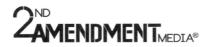

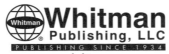

www.whitman.com

© 2015 Whitman Publishing, LLC
3101 Clairmont Road • Suite G • Atlanta, GA 30329

ISBN: 794842674   EAN: 9780794842673

Printed in the United States of America.

CONTENTS

Disclaimer: In a grid-down situation, the world will be much different than the one we know now. Access to medical facilities, medical staff, and medical supplies will be extremely limited or completely unavailable. That is the scenario we write about. Very few of the tips and methods covered in this book should ever be utilized in the world we enjoy now. Most of the procedures herein are extremely dangerous if not performed by a trained medical professional, and we do not advise that any of our readers take this book as an adequate training device to undertake them. Please do not attempt any of these procedures yourself, but instead seek competent care from a licensed medical professional.

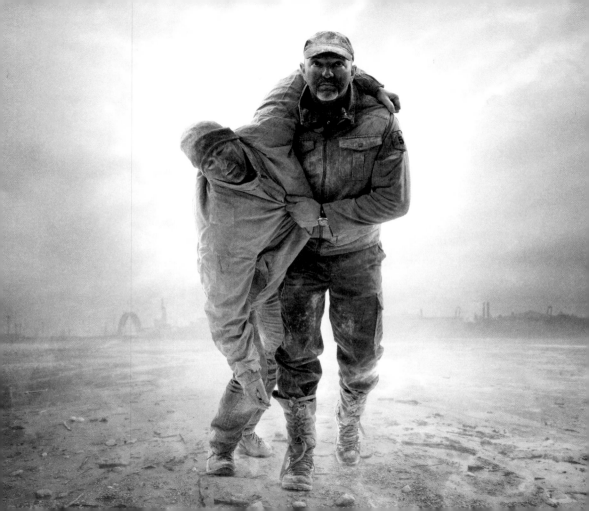

+ INTRODUCTION

Natural disasters, economic crises, terrorist attacks, or any other situation causing a societal breakdown may occur at any time. These situations create difficult circumstances in which proper medical treatment may not be available. Hospitals and emergency medical personnel will not have the ability or resources to treat everyone, especially if the power grid goes down. In these grid-down scenarios, you must rely on your own knowledge and preparations to survive. This book provides helpful tips and recommendations on first aid items and strategies to better equip you and your group during grid-down situations.

Remember: The tips and items recommended in this book are in addition to your current go-bag, vehicle kit, and retreat supplies. The items you choose to include in your medical kits should be tailored to the needs of an individual or group.

 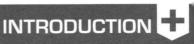

Civilian medical care personnel do not frequently encounter the type of combat trauma a grid-down scenario presents. This book provides you and your medical personnel with relevant guidance on those scenarios. *Grid-Down Survival Guide to First Aid* is your guide to planning, gathering materials, and learning basic knowledge on the management and treatment of medical emergencies in combat-like situations that a disaster scenario may produce. Preparing your gear and gaining personal knowledge gives you a critical advantage in any emergency. Continually conduct further research and training beyond what we offer in the following pages, and apply the knowledge you gain. Knowledge without application is worthless. Practice, train, and rehearse to become proficient and prepared for any unforeseen event.

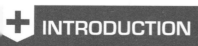

INTRODUCTION

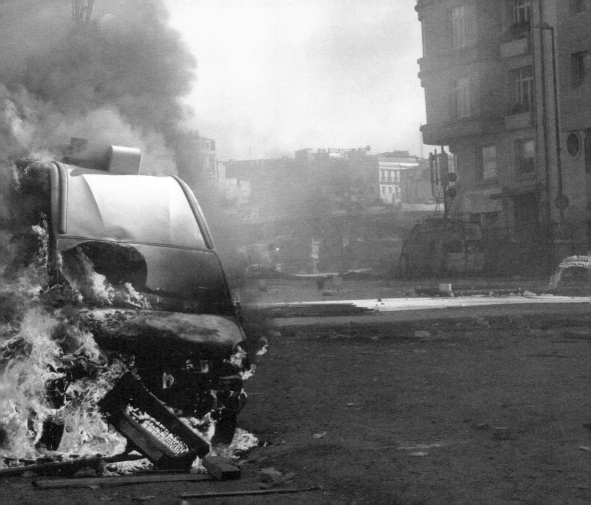

+ PREPARATION

Have your gear ready to go. For proper preparation, you must have your gear staged and ready to go at a moment's notice. You will not have time and likely will not have the money available to purchase everything you need at the last minute. Families and groups must maintain kits for all situations. The guides below give you a great starting point for your kit preparations. You should customize these kits to meet your specific family needs. Even if you purchase pre-packaged first aid kits, you should still customize the contents for yourself or your group. As you customize the kits, familiarize yourself with the contents, understanding where and how to use each item.

Keep your personal aid and individual trauma aid kits readily available at all times. Frequency of use is the distinguishing difference

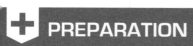

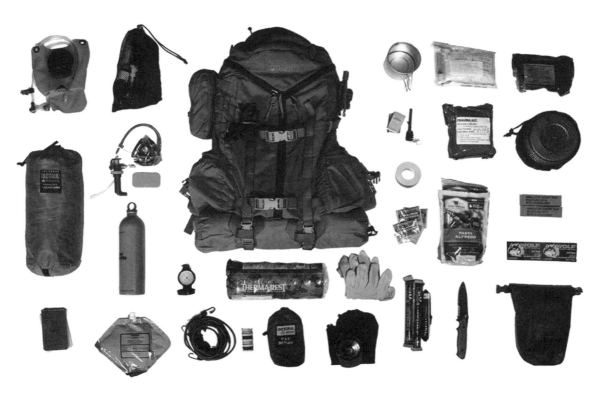

between the two. Personal aid kits (PAK) consist of the basic aid items a person may need on a day-to-day basis. An individual trauma aid kit (ITAK) consists of items for more serious conditions on a longer mission or outing. Terminology may differ as some refer to the trauma kit as an individual first aid kit (IFAK). Either way, keep the personal and trauma kits separate or at least in different compartments, even if you carry both on your person. This will help keep things organized in a time of crisis.

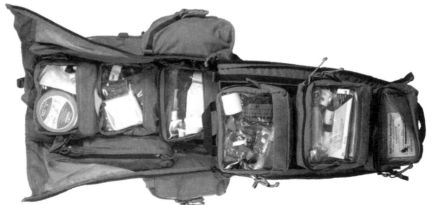

PREPARATION

The Personal Aid Kit (PAK) may consist of:

- Alcohol swabs
- Ibuprofen tablets
- Band-Aids & gauze
- Medical tape
- Antihistamine tablets
- Antiseptic ointment
- Moleskin
- Personal medications
- Antacid tablets
- Water purification tablets

The Individual Trauma Aid Kit (ITAK) should at least consist of the following items:

- Nitrile trauma gloves
- Tourniquet
- Hemostatic gauze
- 4" emergency trauma dressing
- Trauma shears
- Vented chest seal
- Trauma Med (Pill) Pack
- Water purification tablets

 Check with your physician for proper dosage of any medication.

PREPARATION

TRAUMA MED (PILL) PACK

Trauma Med Packs are packages of pre-dosed medications that help fight infection and pain. You will need a prescription to obtain these, but they are worth the hassle to put together.

The military's combat pill pack typically consist of:

- Mobic 15mg—anti-inflamatory
- Tylenol ER 650mg— Acetominophen
- Moxifloxacin/Avelox 400mg— Wide-spectrim antibiotic

 If you have legitimate travel plans to a remote area or you are traveling out of the country, your general care physician should not give you too much of a problem about writing a prescription for these items. Just ask. Be aware of expiration dates.

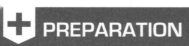 **PREPARATION**

GO-BAG SUPPLEMENTAL KIT

Supplemental item ideas:

- Nasopharyngeal airway 28F with lubricant
- Needle decompression kit
- Z-Fold combat gauze (hemostatic)
- Trauma shears
- Medical tape
- Traction and SAM splints
- Personal medications
- Oropharyngeal airway
- Bag Valve Mask (BVM)

The situation always dictates when and where you store or use each kit. If societal norms remain in effect and you continue in your standard routine of going to work, you probably don't want your personal aid kit and ITAK attached to your belt. So keep them in your go-bag/ready bag or vehicle kit. Just be aware of how heat and cold affects the contents of the kits. When a disaster scenario does occur, always maintain both your personal aid kit and ITAK on your body. Otherwise, you may find that you don't happen to have your kit when you need it. You could also keep a secondary or supplemental set of items in your go-bag or patrol pack.

PREPARATION

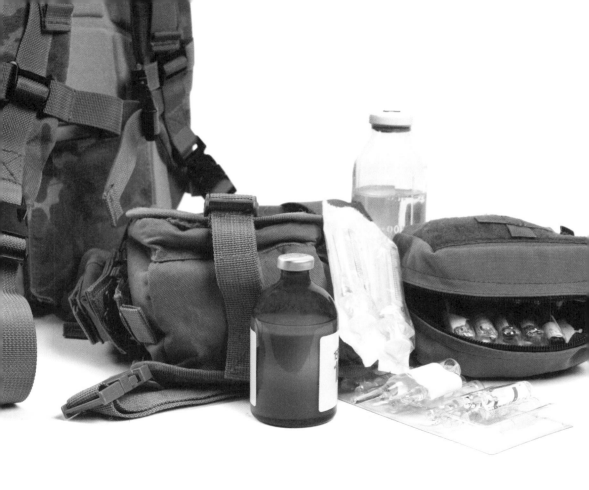

VEHICLE MED KIT

As space, funds, equipment, and situations allow, you will find that having a vehicle med kit is a must in any grid-down survival situation. These kits serve two purposes: supplementing the personal and individual trauma aid kits and helping others. Laying the foundation for long-term survival begins with building trust and health within your immediate area.

Supplemental item ideas:

- Burn dressings
- Water purification devices
- Splint
- Lighting devices
- Casualty evacuation/litter items
- Casualty equipment bag
- Hypothermia prevention items

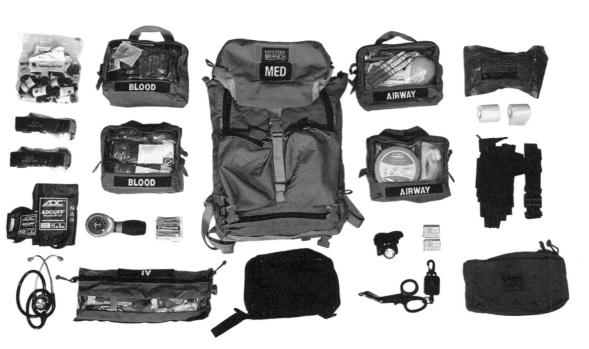

MEDIC KIT

Your individual or group skills should eventually reach the point of advanced medical training. Once you or a member of your group obtains the skills to provide advanced medical treatment, begin investing in more advanced life saving tools. These tools should go into a medic's bag and be worn by the medic at all times.

Items specific to the medic kit include (but are not limited to):

- Sutures
- Nasopharyngeal Airway 28F with lubricant
- Supraglottic airway device
- Tactical suction device
- Needle decompression kit
- Saline lock kit with IV constricting band
- Tactical traction splint
- Medications
- Oral rehydration salts
- Superglue
- SAM Splint

RETREAT KIT

The retreat location needs to be completely stocked, inventoried, and maintained by the group as the triage location—one ready to handle everything from physicals and medication distribution to full—on combat triage care. To do this properly, you will need a dedicated person coordinating the stocking and maintenance of the site. Many of these items should be purchased in large volumes.

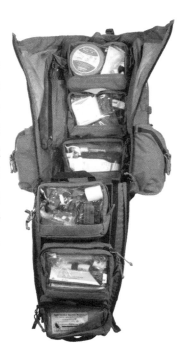

✚ PREPARATION

Recommended items for your retreat location:

- Logbooks/rosters and note taking gear
- Sheets and towels
- Alcohol
- Bleach
- Antibiotics
- Surgical/trauma kit
- Poison control
- Medications and dosage plans
- Rehydration kits
- Sterile saline for IV
- Needeless saline lock kit
- Birthing supplies
- Lice shampoo
- Sanitary napkins
- Toothpaste/antiseptic mouthwash
- Thermometer
- Nail clippers
- Chapstick
- Band-Aids
- Tampons
- Medical tape
- Insect bite/sting relief
- Motrin
- Antibiotic ointment
- Fire starting gear for boiling water

WHEN TO USE KIT CHART

	Normal Day	Hiking/Outdoor Activity	Social Unrest	Bug Out and movement	Retreat work	Post	Patrol	Vehicle Moveme
On Body		Personal Aid	Personal Aid ITAK	Personal Aid ITAK Go-Bag	Personal Aid ITAK	Personal Aid ITAK Go-Bag	Personal Aid ITAK Go-Bag	Personal Ai ITAK
In Vehicle	Personal Aid ITAK	ITAK Vehicle	Go-Bag Vehicle	Vehicle Medic	Vehicle	Vehicle	Vehicle Medic	Vehicle Medic Go-Bag
Staged	Go-Bag Vehicle	Go-Bag	Medic Retreat	Retreat	Go-Bag Medic Retreat	Medic Retreat	Retreat	Retreat
Stored	Medic Retreat	Medic Retreat						

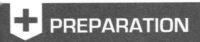

PREPARATION

GROUP TRAINING

Regardless of how much money your group has spent on supplies or how many books and blogs you have read, your group is not adequately prepared for a grid-down situation until you've invested personal and group time into training. Every individual of classroom age should undergo training to utilize the medical equipment within your inventory. Some excellent training classes are offered by the Red Cross, EMT certification centers, and community colleges. However, the ideal training is scenario-based training. A company called ArmorCorps, based out of Tennessee, provides basic scenario based trauma care training at a very reasonable price. Their training differs from most in that it is a live-fire, overnight, combat casualty care, scenario-based training that recreates the stress of a grid-down firefight situation. You will learn how to train other individuals within your group in CPR, wound packing/dressing, burn dressing/care, suturing, and the Four Lifesaving Steps. Classes like this are great "hip-pocket" classes that allow members to refine and maintain their skills by having to train others.

Group training doesn't stop with educational training on process or treatment. Group training also consists of physical fitness training. Moving a casualty out of harm's way takes endurance, brute force, and pure muscle. Don't think that adrenaline is going to be your source of muscle. People who think they will lift cars by their own strength prompted by an extreme stressor like a desire to save their little ones will quickly realize this logic doesn't apply in situations requiring tremendous amounts of energy to be exerted over an extended period. Overeating, consumption of processed junk food, and lack of exercise can be fatal if a grid-down situation occurs. Individuals who are not in shape will have trouble contributing to the team equally. If you can't quickly ascend a flight of stairs while carrying your go-bag without shortness of breath, then you are not in proper physical shape.

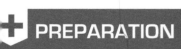

PREPARATION

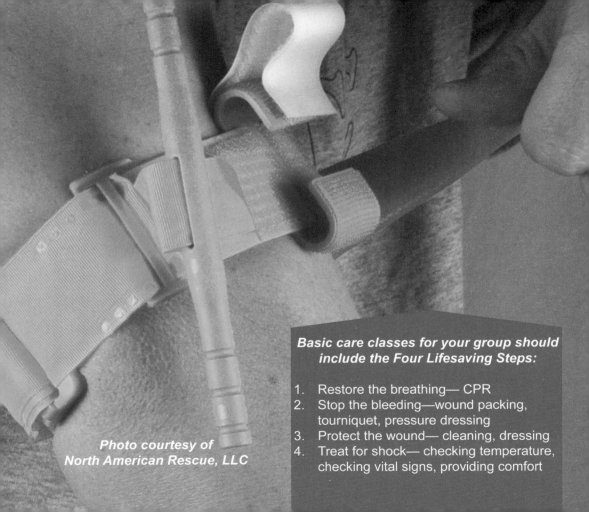

Basic care classes for your group should include the Four Lifesaving Steps:

1. Restore the breathing— CPR
2. Stop the bleeding—wound packing, tourniquet, pressure dressing
3. Protect the wound— cleaning, dressing
4. Treat for shock— checking temperature, checking vital signs, providing comfort

Photo courtesy of North American Rescue, LLC

+ PREVENTION

The absolute best method for protecting your wellbeing or that of your group or family is to prevent injury or sickness. The prevention of injury and sickness comes in the form of lifestyle, knowledge, and gear. Change your lifestyle today to match that of a grid-down environment. This will instill good

Sanitation plans should include:

- Trash
- Food waste
- Human waste
- Wound care waste
- Medical tool sanitation
- Death and biohazard disposal

habits into the group. As a group or family leader, you must consider the health and human needs of your community. Realize that many things relate to healthcare and that you need to consider your group's needs during the preparation phase. The balance between prevention and treatment is a decision you will have to make at every level. The limited

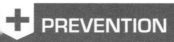

PREVENTION

supply of medicine forces reasonable use, while limited access to healthcare will force proper training and teaching. Prior to the occurrence of a disaster situation and thereafter, monitor your local resources to help make decisions on what to do and when to take action.

A key part of prevention is proper sanitation. Individual hygiene is critical to personal and group health and must not be neglected. Simply washing your hands plays a huge role in maintaining good health. Always wash your hands before and after using the bathroom, preparing food, handling livestock, sleeping, assisting with injuries, helping the ill, handling food stores, and any situation where people gather.

DENTAL HYGIENE

Dental Hygiene during a grid-down situation is just as crucial to healthy living as washing your hands. Imagine trying to find a dentist during a collapse. Stay current on your dental checkups prior to any grid-down situation. Don't get complacent after a hard day's work—brush and floss your teeth. Strong, healthy teeth are necessary if you want to stay alive in a grid-down situation. Cavities are not easily fixed and can cause severe pain, while decayed or rotten teeth can lead to serious infections.

Dental Tips:

Always stock extra toothbrushes, toothpaste, and antiseptic mouthwash. If you don't have a toothbrush available, clean your teeth using twigs sharpened at one end and chewed at the other. You can also tie a rough piece of towel to the end of a stick to create a toothbrush. If you don't

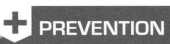

PREVENTION

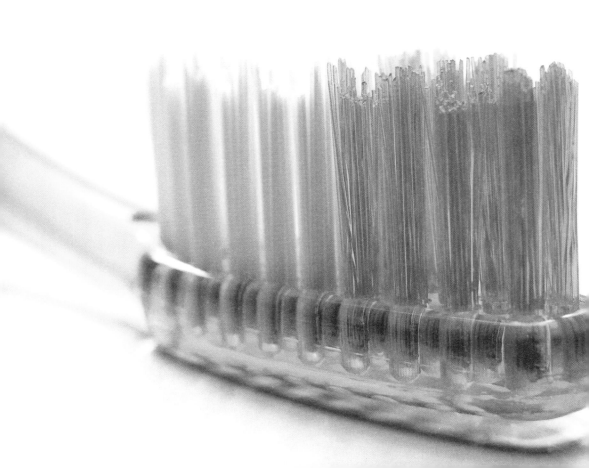

have toothpaste, simply extend the time you spend brushing your teeth with just water. If you want to make a paste, mix salt and baking soda then add a bit of water. Use caution if you utilize hydrogen peroxide when brushing as many dentists report that this may cause a breakdown of enamel. Keep a crown replacement kit at your retreat location.

TAKING CARE OF YOUR FEET

It is important to realize how much time you will likely spend on your feet in a grid-down scenario and how important they are to your ability to contribute to your family and group. Take care of them by purchasing proper footwear and be sure your shoes are the correct size. DO NOT oversize your shoe/boot for comfort, as extra room allows your foot to move within the shoe, creating blisters. If you ask a legitimate shoe-fitting professional, they will tell you all too often, that men think they

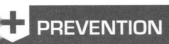

PREVENTION

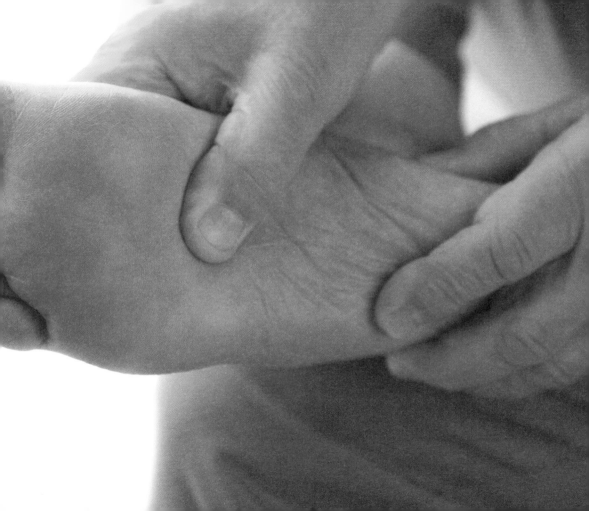

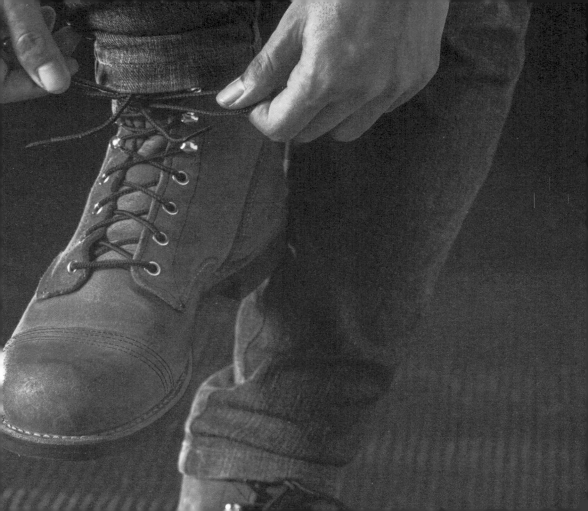

wear a size that is at least one size too big. Invest in proper footwear for your conditions/climate, and replace your worn or improperly fitted footwear immediately. When preparing for a long day's work or extended foot movement, always pack an extra pair of socks. When sleeping, do not sleep in your shoes. Allow your feet to breathe, keeping them cool. Avoid putting on wet socks at all costs. Trim your toenails and keep them clean. By keeping your feet cool and moisture free and reducing friction, you will do much to reduce foot injury and infection due to blisters. Even if you can't take a shower at the end of the day, remove your boots and wash your feet. Let them dry to help prevent sores. Utilize moleskin to ward off blisters.

Important Tip:
In a grid-down scenario, you may encounter nails, glass, and other debris that could penetrate the soles of your shoes or boots. Prepare for this by purchasing boots with a steel or composite shank.

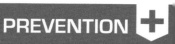

PREVENTION

PROTECTIVE CLOTHING

Don't neglect the importance of dressing for the occasion. If you're going to be out chopping wood and clearing brush, then wear heavy pants, boots, a long-sleeved shirt, a hat, protective glasses, gloves and bug spray. EVERY one of these items will play a tremendous role in preventing injury. However, you must actually wear them. Do not think, "Oh, I'm only doing a little bit of work today so I don't need to fool with that." This sort of complacency will get you killed in a long-term grid-down situation. Knee and elbow pads also provide excellent protection and comfort. Layer clothing for varying temperatures and conditions.

HYDRATE

If you do not hydrate, you will die. One of the easiest ways to check for proper hydration is to observe the color of your urine. Clear to pale-yellow urine indicates that you are properly hydrated, whereas dark

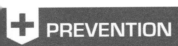

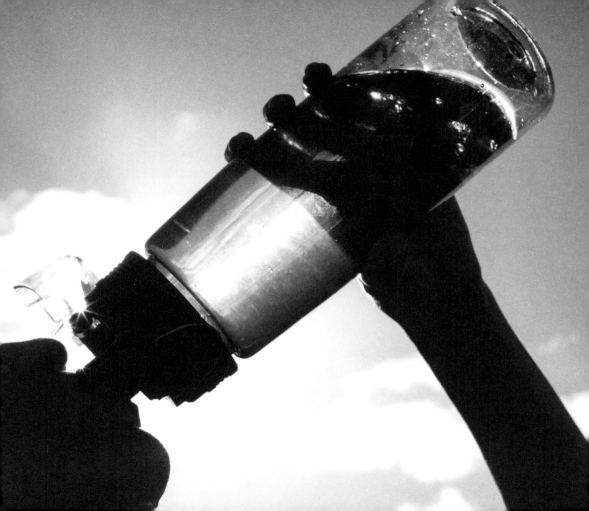

yellow signals dehydration. Always make sure you're drinking safe water when hydrating by boiling or using filters or chemical treatments. Just be careful not to overdo the consumption of chemically-treated water. The best way to do this is by utilizing MSR AquaTabs. They are one of the few chemical tabs approved for extended consumption of treated water. While preparing for survival situations, it is a good idea to purchase items like hydration packs or bags. MSR also makes a very rugged Hydromedary bladder with a drink tube. Having the drink tube right at your mouth encourages frequent hydration. In a survival situation, drink at least one gallon of water per day.

IMMUNIZATIONS

Vaccines help protect against diseases. Depending on your area and personal views, vaccinations can begin as soon as birth and often require several treatments to achieve effectiveness. Thus, if you want to receive vaccinations, know your treatment process and schedule. Speak to your

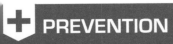

PREVENTION

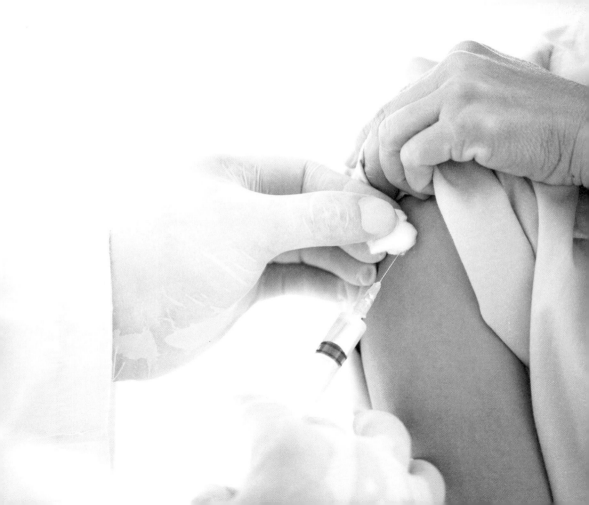

healthcare provider and have them spend time working out a personal schedule. Don't allow them to gloss over the topic because they simply follow a government prescribed schedule. Know what you're getting and when you're getting it. Inspect packaging to ensure the contents are the proper vaccination prior to any application. Bring your schedule with you to the clinic. Most vaccines are given as an infant or child, but many may be given as an adult. Consult your physician for what is best for you.

Some of the most common vaccines include:

- Tetanus, diphtheria, and pertussis (Td/Tdap)
- Polio
- Smallpox
- Diphtheria
- Varicella—chickenpox
- Typhoid
- Malaria
- Rabies
- BCG/tuberculosis
- MMR—measles, mumps, rubella
- Hepatitis A
- Hepatitis B
- Haemophilos influensae (Hib)
- Rotavirus

PREVENTION

COMMONLY STOCKED MEDICATIONS
Over the Counter—OTC

OTC meds can be used to treat many issues resulting from or magnified by a grid-down situation. OTC meds can be used to effectively treat or minimize the effects of many conditions such as heartburn, ulcers, diarrhea, allergies, nausea, vomiting, eczema, hives, earache, sore throat, fever, headache, menstrual cramps, arthritis, insomnia,

Common OTC meds:

- Pseudoephedrine (Sudafed)
- Loperamide (Imodium)
- Meclizine (Bonine, Dramamine)
- Acetaminophen (Tylenol)
- Ibuprofen (Motrin, Advil)
- Ranitidine (Zantac)
- Clotrimazole (Gyne-Lotrimin)
- Hydrocortisone cream
- Bacitracin ointment

diaper rash, and many others. Use this list as a starting point or collection list. If you do not have these meds on hand by the time a disaster strikes, make sure your group members know to be on the lookout for any medications available.

PREVENTION

PRESCRIPTION MEDICATIONS

Obviously, any prescription you are currently taking needs to be be stockpiled for as long as possible and an rotated regularly. Other prescription medications, such as antibiotics, can come in very handy when no hospital treatment is available.

Common Prescription Medications:

- Ciprofloxacin (Cipro) 500mg
- Azithromycin 250mg
- Amoxicillin 500mg
- Trimethoprim-sulfamethoxazole 160mg/800mg
- Doxycycline 100mg
- Metronidazole 500mg
- Cephalexin 500mg
- Clindamycin 300mg

Notice: This is a list of commonly recommended medications. You should seek proper knowledge, training, and guidance from a licensed medical physician prior to treating any condition. Serious complications can occur due to the misuse of these treatments and medications.

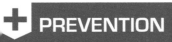

PREVENTION

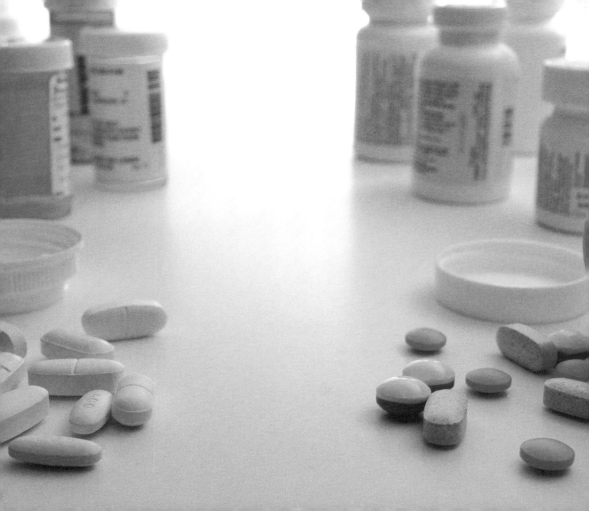

KEEPING YOUR MEDICATIONS AND WATER COOL

A very popular method of keeping items cool is the "pot-in-pot" assembly. This method dates back thousands of years. It can be used to keep medications cool or keep water cool for heat casualties.

POT-IN-POT QUICK INSTRUCTIONS

You will need:

- 2 clay pots (one pot should nicely fit inside the other)
- Sand
- Towel
- Water

PREVENTION

Step one: Plug any holes in the pots

Step two: Place small amount of sand in bottom of larger pot—just enough sand to make the top of the smaller pot level with the top of the larger pot when placed inside

Step three: Place smaller pot inside larger pot

Step four: Fill the outer void between the two pots with sand

Step five: Saturate sand with water

Final step: Cover with wet towel

Effects: In a shaded area this low cost low energy method of cooling will keep its contents 25-60% cooler than ambient temperatures.

Benefit: Keeps medications, water, fruit, and vegetables cool.

Warnings: The internal temperature of the pots may fluctuate in certain environments. The constant fluctuation of temperature may be more harmful to medications than a constant temperature of an underground storage unit such as a root cellar. Also, water used in this process of cooling creates a high-humidity environment inside the chambers.

PREVENTION

+ TREATMENT

INITIAL ASSESSMENT:

Assess the Situation

Prior to assessing the wounded, assess the area! Find out if the scene is safe. Accidents and casualties tend to multiply. Ensure that the area is secure from hostiles and that your team has established firepower superiority and set up a 360-degree perimeter. Look for immediate hazards in the area if the injury is accidental. This includes avoiding rock falls or an avalanche and goes as far as ensuring you have proper clothing and equipment as the rescuer. Then, if necessary and possible without causing additional injury, move the casualty to a safe area for treatment. In a combat situation, you may have to move the casualty while taking fire. Remember to return fire and elimate the threat before treating or moving a casualty.

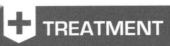

TREATMENT

Check the Breathing

Check the casualty's airway for signs of breathing. If the patient can speak, the airway is generally clear. If they are unconscious, place your ear next to his/her nose and listen or feel for air movement. If there is no air movement, then check for obstructions such as the tongue. Provide CPR if there is no air movement.

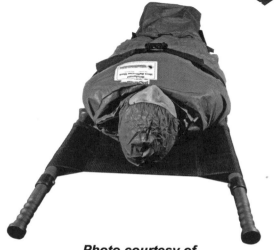

Photo courtesy of
North American Rescue, LLC

Check Circulation

If the victim does not have a pulse, begin CPR.

TREATMENT ✚

Check for Bleeding

Conduct a quick check for severe blood loss visually and with your hands.

Check for Spinal Injury

During the initial assessment, keep the back and neck as still as possible. This is especially important in fall or head trauma cases.

CUTS, SCRAPES, AND WOUNDS

During a grid-down situation, your survival will depend greatly on your ability to utilize your personal aid kit and apply self-treatment when working or on a patrol. For small cuts, scrapes, and gaping wounds, use the supplies in your personal aid and individual trauma aid kit to clean, protect, and promote healing.

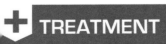 **TREATMENT**

First, clean the area. Using alcohol pads, antiseptic wipes, or a sterile wash, remove debris from the wound. In the case of a gaping wound, pack the wound with sterile saline soaked gauze and apply pressure. Within reason, allow the initial flow of blood to wash out debris and bacteria. However, for obvious and life-threatening blood loss, stop the bleeding immediately. Generally, you can stop the bleeding by applying pressure. Pressure may have to be applied for an extended period of time. If the wound is on an arm or leg, raising the extremity above the heart will slow the bleeding. If the blood soaks through the gauze, apply more gauze and continue applying pressure. If the bleeding will not stop, apply a tourniquet. When cleaning lacerations, forcefully flush the wound with clean water. Ideally, use a needle-less or irrigating syringe for cleaning. This will remove foreign matter and debris. Cleaning the wound is a painful process. Ideally, clean as quickly as possible. This will not only reduce the risk of infection, but will also reduce the amount and duration of pain to the casualty.

TREATMENT ✚

Large lacerations require closure. You can close the wound using several methods, including tape, sutures, and staples. Just as with small wounds, allowing them to bleed momentarily will encourage the release of bacteria and debris from the wound. If the bleeding is profuse, apply direct pressure. One method is to tape

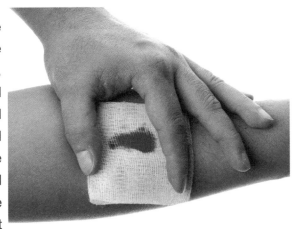

the wound shut using butterfly bandages, which are readily available in most first aid kits. If you do not have butterfly bandages available, you can make them by using small strips of tape and nonstick gauze. However, this method is not sterile.

TREATMENT

Sutures are available in many options. The skill of the applicator and the area needing sutures determines the method of suturing to use. 3-0 nylon sutures with pre-attached curved needles are ideal for closing lacerations with a lot of tension, such as the back, scalp, or scapular areas. For most other lacerations without excessive tension, 4-0 nlylon sutures work well. They typically come in sterile packets ready to use. In order to use these sutures, you will need to practice and have necessary tools, such as scissors and a needle holder, readily availablle. Work with a nurse, medic, or doctor to learn how to properly suture as this can take some time to master.

Stapling is a fast and easy way to close a gaping laceration. Disposable staplers and staple removers are readily available and fairly inexpensive. They also require little to no training, assuming the use of a little common sense. Stapling can significantly reduce wound closure time and the visible scarring is nearly identical to monofilament sutures.

In an emergency, many people use Super Glue to close small wounds. Many doctors advise that Super Glue works well in a pinch, but may cuse irritation in some cases, as it is not a medical grade product. Several medical approved skin adhesives exist, such as Dermabond or SurgiSeal, but can be expensive.

BURNS

Quickly remove the source of heat from a casualty. Smother any flames quickly and cleanly. Submerse in cool (not cold) clean water for 10-15 minutes to eliminate debris getting into the burn area. Do not use direct ice and do not submerse burns covering a large portion of the body in cool water for too long due to risk of hypothermia. Be sure not to over cool any victim, as shock is common in burn situations. Assess the type of burn to determine if it is 1st, 2nd, or 3rd degree.

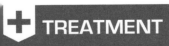

TREATMENT

1st degree burns typically result from light scalding or sunburn. Some swelling and reddening around the burn may occur. In the event of 1st degree burns, the casualty typically won't need to be removed from the effort. In most cases, the pain will subside after about 24 hours. As long as the burn only covers a small portion of the body, most casualties can take ibuprofen from their personal aid kit and keep working.

The 3 types of burns:

- 1st degree—Only the first layer of skin is burned.
- 2nd degree—Two layers of skin are burned.
- 3rd degree—All three layers of skin are burned and may have deeper burns into tissue or bone are possible.

TREATMENT

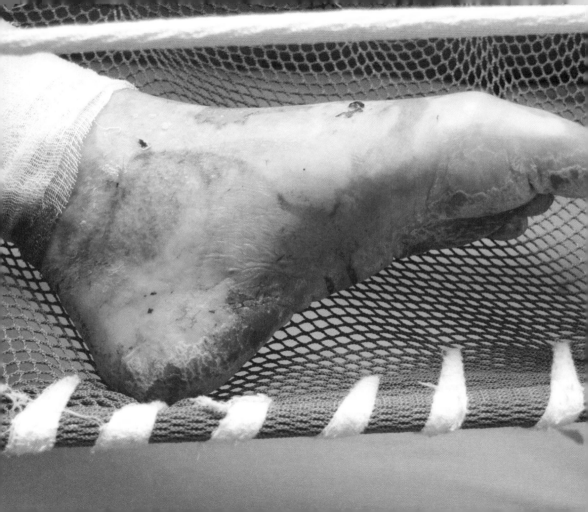

2nd degree burns occur when a very hot object or boiling water burns through two layers of skin. Sunburn can also cause 2nd degree burns. Cover the burn area with soft but non-fibrous gauze and apply antibiotic ointment if the skin is broken.

In the case of 2nd degree burns of less than 15% of the body area or 3rd degree burns of less than 10% of the body area, clean the area with surgical scrub or non-medicated soap. Use caution if attempting to remove debris stuck in the wound

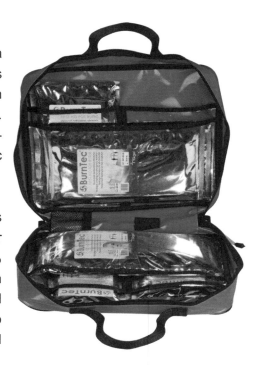

TREATMENT ✚

area as this can cause further damage. The use of burn dressings is best in this situation. Hydrogel dressings are common as they provide up to 24-hour soothing effects, are impermeable to bacteria, and reduce scarring. 3rd degree burns larger than a fifty cent piece (3cm) will require a skin graft to heal properly.

3rd degree burns greater than 10% and 2nd degree burns greater than 15% will require immediate evacuation from the area. Burn care in this situation should be focused on keeping the wound clean, reducing the pain, and treating for shock. In order to treat for shock you must keep the casualty adequately hydrated. Push as much fluid as the casualty can hold down. Vomiting will increase the risk of dehydration. If the patient falls into a coma, provide fluids intravenously. Provide medication for the pain as the situation allows. By the third day, start a high carbohydrate food plan with substantial amounts of protein and vitamins. If available, provide multivitamins every day.

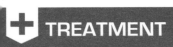

TREATMENT

FRACTURES

Bone fractures will likely increase during a grid-down survival situation due to extreme increases in outdoor work and hard labor. Moving sandbags, digging fighting holes, and moving logs can all contribute to the increased risk. A fracture simply means a bone has been broken. Do not rely on restricted movement to diagnose a fracture. There are several types of fractures, and some are not easily identifiable by perceived pain during movement. Use point tenderness and obvious pain to identify the presence of a fracture. Many first aid courses cover splinting extensively. It is highly recommended that you take those courses and practice splinting.

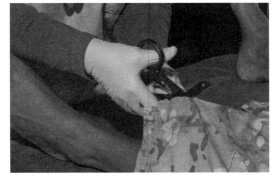

TREATMENT ➕

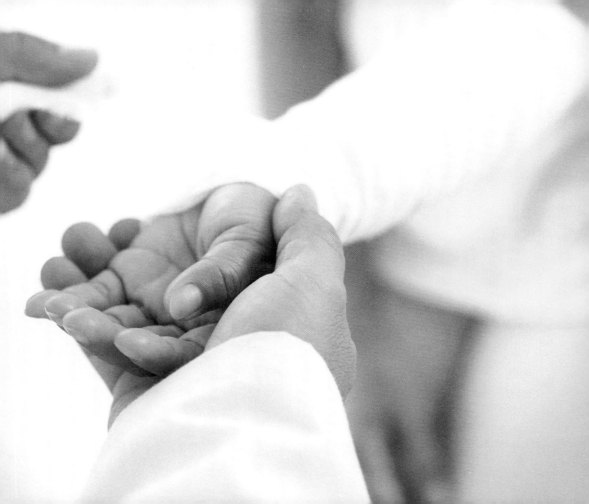

Many classes will teach you splint in place until you can get an x-ray. However, that technique only helpful when a hospital is only minutes away. In a grid-down situation, you will want to use gentle traction to realign the break prior to splinting. Extremely angulated fractures can cause the veins to bend which reduces the flow of blood to the extremity. By realigning, you will open those veins and allow blood flow to return. By observing and comparing the pulse on the opposite extremity, you will more easily determine

Some key points to remember when diagnosing and treating fractures.

1) Circulation and nerve damage caused by deformity should be corrected.
2) Prevent infection by cleaning the area around an open fracture or wound near a fracture.
3) Prevent tissue damage by using a well-padded splint.
4) Align the fracture for proper healing.

TREATMENT

proper flow than if you were to merely evaluate the side with the break. Risk of damaging the veins is rather low, but always use caution when providing traction to the fracture. In the event of an open fracture or wound near a fracture, irrigate and clean the area. After proper cleaning, cover the area with triple antibiotic ointment. The risk of a serious bone infection is extremely high if the area is not cleaned properly. Once cleaned and prepped, soak sterile dressings in sterile water and apply over the open wound. Then apply and secure a dry dressing over the wet dressing. Change twice daily. During the recovery, the area below or around the fracture may bruise, swell, or discolor.

CPR

Cardiopulmonary Resuscitation (CPR) is an emergency lifesaving procedure designed to circulate oxygen through the lungs and blood through the heart. This will provide partial flow of oxygenated blood

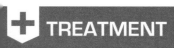

TREATMENT

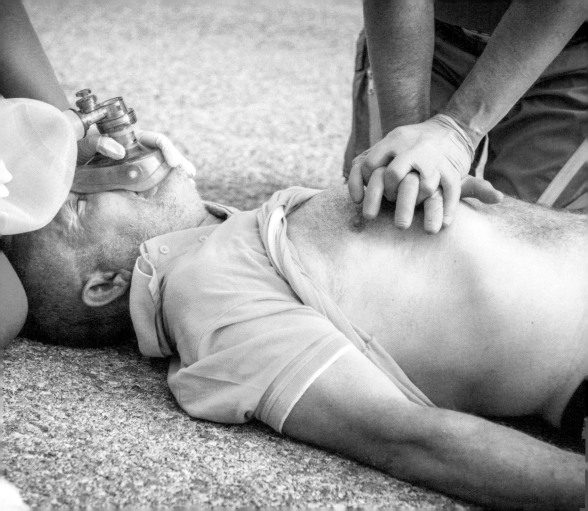

to the brain. Many organizations provide CPR classes at a relatively inexpensive cost and it is highly recommended to attend these courses.

Apply CPR after the area secure and you have assessed that the person is not breathing. After positioning the casualty flat on their back, there are two simple steps to remember.

If two rescuers are present, provide the breaths without pause in compression at a rate of one breath

CPR Steps:

Step 1: Compress—the adult chest at a rate of at least 100 compressions per minute with a compression depth of at least 2 inches. The rescuer should allow complete recoil of the chest after each compression, to allow the heart to fill completely before the next compression.

Step 2: Provide mouth-to-mouth—tilt the head back enough to lift the chin and pinch the nose. Provide full breaths and deliver over one full second. Give two breaths after every 30 conpressions (a 30:2 compression to ventilation ratio)

TREATMENT

every 6 to 8 seconds (8 to 10 ventilations per mnute). Death is almost certainly the outcome if you do not provide CPR to an unconscious victim who is not breathing and does not have an identifiable pulse.

COLD WEATHER CASUALTIES

Hypothermia

Hypothermia medically refers to the core temperature of a person dropping below 95°, which is only a 3.6° drop below normal. When the core temperature drops below 90°, this causes moderate hypothermia. Temperatures below 82° are considered severe. Do not be fooled into thinking that you can only develop hypothermia in extreme cold environments. Even in mild weather, you can develop hypothermia. Any blood loss can also contribute to hypothermia.

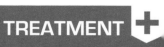

TREATMENT

During a survival situation, you may face three types of hypothermia:

- **Acute or immersion**—rapid heat loss, typically onset by immersion in water
- **Chronic**—heat loss over time, typically onset by inadequate clothing
- **Exhaustion**—heat loss caused by extreme physical exertion where the body can no longer produce heat

Prevent hypothermia by ensuring each member of your group or family is in good physical condition. Hydration, proper nutrition, and adequate clothing greatly reduce the risk of hypothermia. Dress in layers that are easily removed and reapplied so that you don't increase the dampness of your clothing. Damp clothes will increase the evaporative cooling effect. You must stay dry. During an extended period of cold weather, a group can use each other's body heat to stay warm. When exhaustion is not present, rapid exercise will dramatically increase body temperature.

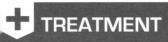

TREATMENT

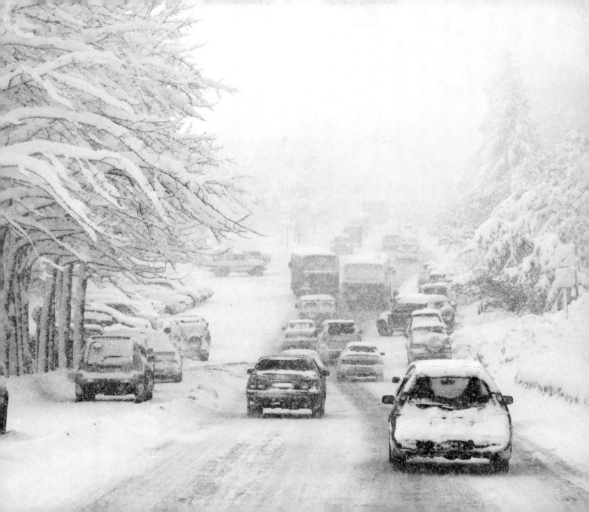

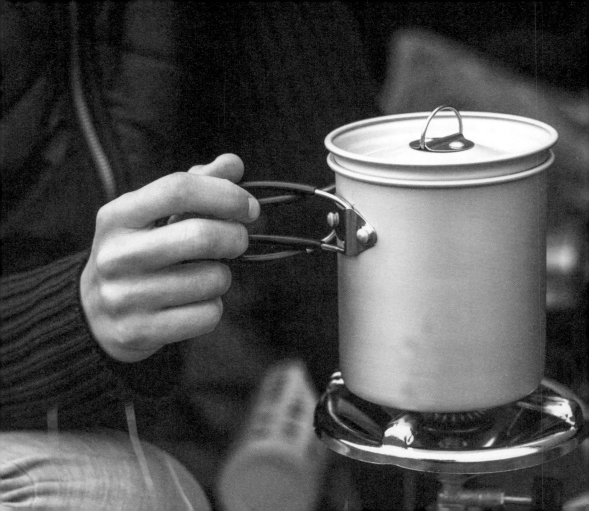

Treating hypothermia requires preventing further heat loss by removing any wet clothing and replacing with dry clothing. A hypothermia kit containing reflective blankets and skullcaps will greatly increase treatment effectiveness. The quickest way to overcome hypothermia is to drink warm liquids. Remember, it is much easier to prevent hypothermia than it is to treat.

Types of cold weather injuries include:

- Chilblains
- Immersion Foot (trench foot)
- Frostnip and Frostbite

Cold weather injuries must be taken very seriously as they can be life threatening without hospitals or doctors in close proximity. Take precautions and prepare yourself to help eliminate or greatly reduce the risk of injury. Primarily ensure you remain in peak physical condition. Wear proper clothing and layers to insulate. Stay dry and change your socks frequently.

Chilblains

Chilblains occur when dry skin is exposed to temperatures below 60° F to freezing. The skin will itch and be red, swollen and sometimes tender. The best treatment is prevention. Prevent exposed skin by staying covered even if by only a light fabric just to keep the wind off the skin. If you have petroleum jelly or hydrocortisone, you can apply as needed to help the healing process.

Immersion Foot

Immersion foot (also known as trench foot) is caused primarily by exposure of the feet to cool/cold, wet conditions. This injury is extremely serious. In the preliminary stages of immersion foot, the foot shows swelling, develops dark spots, and remains cold and seemingly waxy. Due to a lack of feeling in the foot, walking becomes difficult. The progression into the next stage leads to hot, swollen, and red feet.

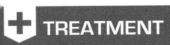

TREATMENT

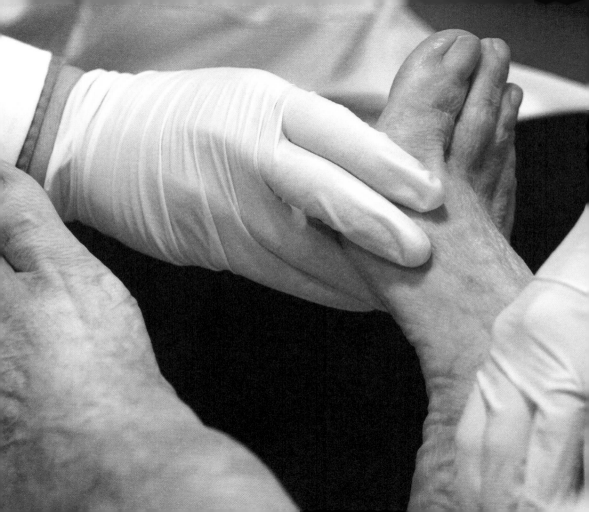

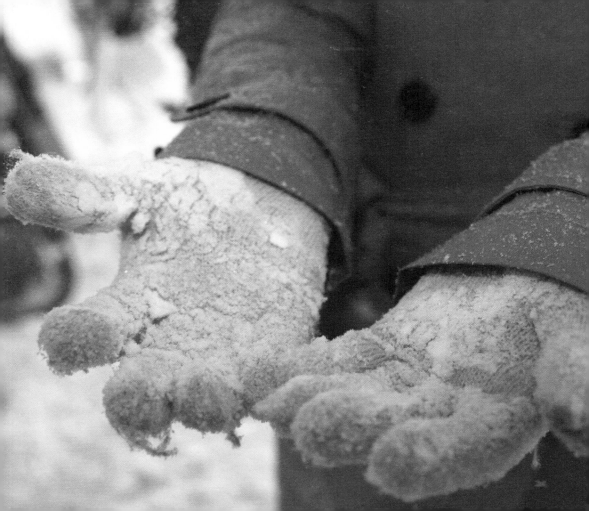

Blisters will form and are typically the cause of infection and gangrene. Reduce your risk of immersion foot by frequently changing your socks. At the very least, remove your socks every night. To treat immersion foot, reduce the bloods ability to clot by taking aspirin. Take pain medication as needed. Increase the blood flow to the feet as well as possible.

Frostnip & Frostbite

Frostnip is the beginning stages of frostbite of the superficial tissue. It can affect people differently even within the same environment or group. Typically, frostnip affects the tip of the nose and the edges of the ears. You will see the skin turn white, and you must recognize and catch it quickly enough to apply warmth and thaw the area thoroughly.

Frostbite is the complete freezing and destruction of the skin tissue. Temperatures below freezing, inadequate insulation, and circulation are the primary causes of frostbite. Be cautious of tight clothing and boots and even diseases such as diabetes that affect blood vessels.

Treatment can be conducted using two methods, passive and active rewarming. Passive rewarming consists of removing the affected area from the cold and insulating properly. Whereas active rewarming is the application of direct heat. Soaking the area in water at 104° to 108° will quickly thaw the frozen area. The quicker you can thaw and treat the area the better. Just be sure the risk of refreezing is low. The formation of ice crystals can severely damage the cells. For that reason, do not attempt to rub or handle a frostbite area. Splint the area properly and avoid movement as much as possible.

HEAT CASUALTIES

Heat and dehydration can cause three major heat casualties: heat cramps, heat exhaustion, and heat stroke. Other less severe heat casualties include sunburn and prickly heat.

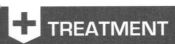

TREATMENT

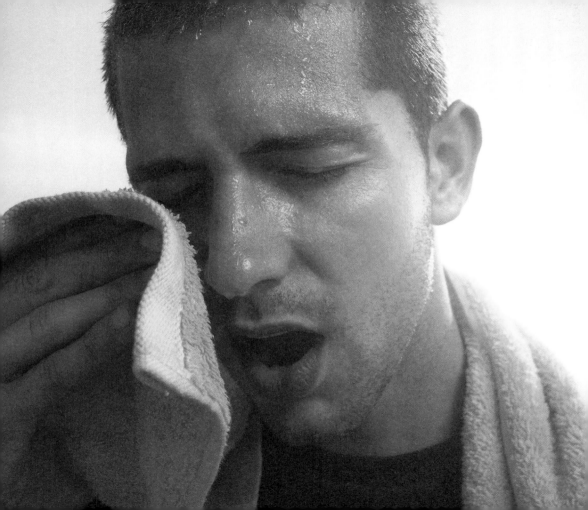

Prevention: proper fluid intake, proper clothing, proper diet, and physical fitness.

Heat cramps are typically caused by the depletion of salt during intense activity, specifically in hot environments. Treat by resting, consuming salty foods, and hydrating with electrolyte enhanced fluids if possible.

Heat exhaustion is quite simply shock due to hot environments. It is the most common heat illness typically developed over several days and is a result of the body needing more blood flow than the cardiovascular system can manage. The casualty will be pale in color and will experience a rapid heart rate, nausea, headache, dizziness, and lightheadedness.

Treating for heat exhaustion is similar to treating for shock. Reduce the labor of the heart by cooling the body and allowing it to rest. Remove clothing and place the casualty in shade. Quickly get the person to drink as much water as they can handle. Rehydration mix is recommended.

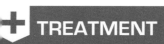 **TREATMENT**

Heat stroke, sometimes referred to as sun stroke, is the complete breakdown of bodily thermal regulation. Casualties loose the ability to sweat and their core temperature could rise over 105° and as high as 115°, causing a severe emergency. Immediately move the casualty to a shaded area and cool with any means possible. Remove clothing, fan, and soak or spray the casualty with water. Keep the casualty hydrated and in stable temperatures for as long as necessary. The person's body, even after regaining consciousness, may not be able to regulate temperature effectively.

Sunburn is common but shouldn't be overlooked. The discomfort sunburns cause can severely distract anyone working or trying to stay vigilant while on post. Treat these burns just as you would a 1st degree burn.

Although not as well known, prickly heat is a rash caused by the glands of the skin trapping a person's sweat. This can affect mental focus. Cool the person, dry the area, and avoid further sweating.

TREATMENT

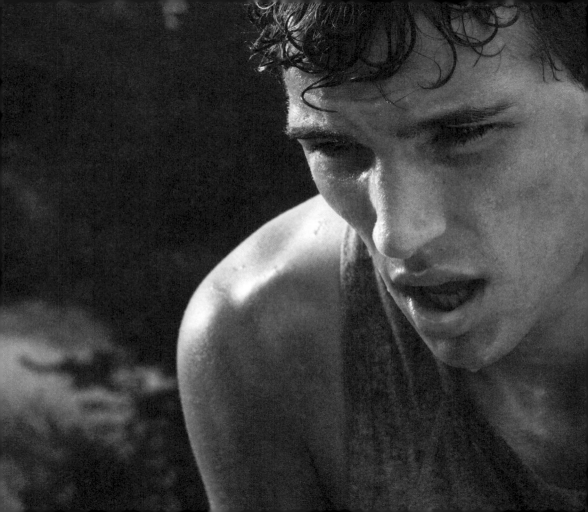

DEHYDRATION

Dehydration occurs when the body loses more fluid than it takes in. Extreme physical exertion over extended periods causes sweat or evaporation of liquids. Dehydration can also ensue as a result of diarrhea or vomiting. When a person is extremely ill and cannot take in food or fluid, dehydration is a major concern. Urine should stay clear or at least a pale yellow. Remember that dehydration is not limited to high heat areas. Dehydration can occur in any environment.

Signs of dehydration include:

- Thirst and dry mouth
- Feeling lightheaded
- Little or no urine; urine is dark in color
- Loss of skin elasticity
- Sunken eyes, usually tearless
- Infants may have sunken soft spots

TREATMENT ✚

Severe dehydration can mask itself as shock. Fast but weak pulse, fever, and deep breathing can all be symptoms of dehydration.

Act rapidly to prevent dehydration. Drink as much water as possible while consuming normal amounts of food. A rehydration drink is best for preventing and treating dehydration. A homemade oral re-hydration salt (ORS) mix consists of 1 liter of water, ½ teaspoon of salt, and 6 teaspoons of sugar. Consume as much rehydration mix as possible without inducing vomiting. A larger person should consume as much as 3 liters per day.

✚ TREATMENT

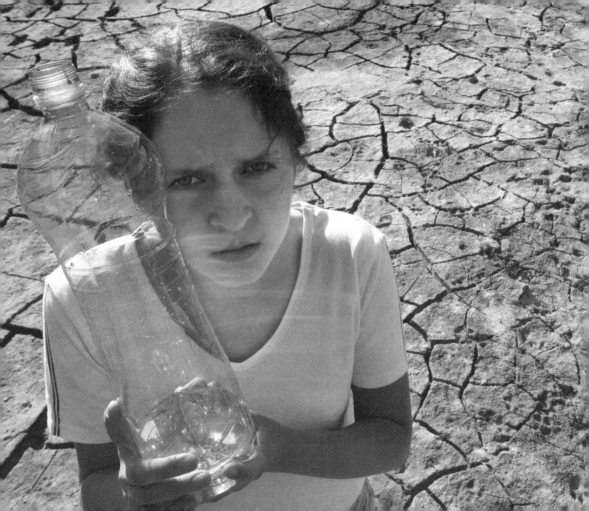

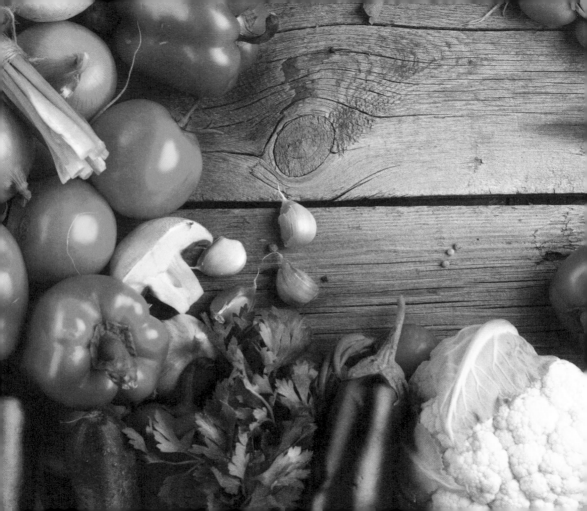

MALNUTRITION

A diet lacking a balance of nutrients causes malnutrition. In a survival situation, many experts advise maintaining a well balanced diet consisting of proteins, carbohydrates, fruits, and especially dark green leafy vegetables. A stock of whole food vitamins often helps maintain essential nutrients.

Effects of malnutrition range greatly, but can result in:

- Weakness and muscle loss
- Anemia
- Wounds healing slowly
- Scurvy
- Sores around the mouth
- Low immune response

The most important aspect to remember is that proper nutrition helps to fight sickness. Food production should be your utmost concern after water and the defense of your family or group.

SEIZURES

Seizures vary in type and seriousness. Illness, drugs, head injuries, heat illness, fever, or low blood sugar can cause seizures. The most serious and recognizable seizure is a grand mal or full body seizure. They can last between 2-3 minutes and cause other injuries due to falling or convulsive movements into hard objects. Address the episode by removing surrounding objects and allowing the person to move freely. Make sure the airway is clear and do not put anything in the person's mouth. Roll the casualty on his or her side to help keep them from choking. If the person loses unconsciousness and stops breathing, begin CPR.

ASTHMA

Asthma can be a life-threatening respiratory disease involving the bronchial tubes. Pollen, foods, respiratory infections, stress, exercise, and even exposure to cold air can make a person susceptible to an attack.

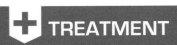 **TREATMENT**

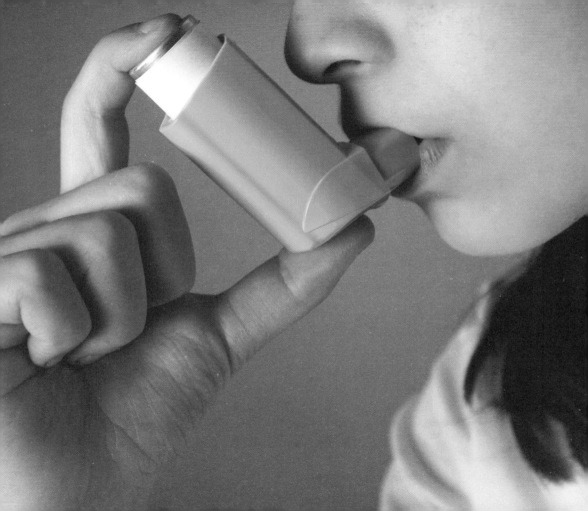

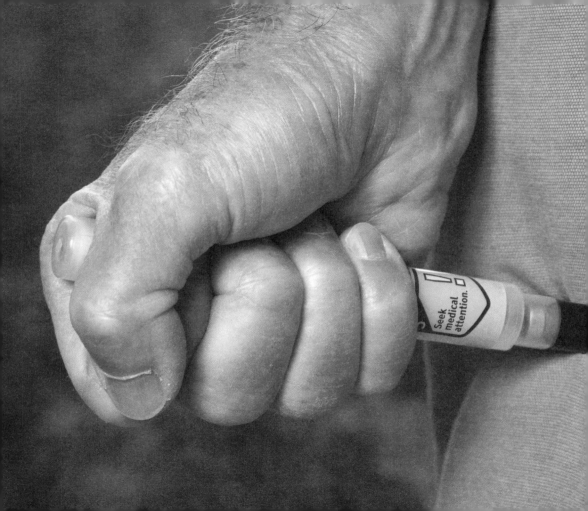

Signs or symptoms of an acute attack are wheezing, coughing, and the feeling of not getting enough air. This is due to muscles around the breathing tubes in the lungs constricting. Breathing medications and inhalers are the most common forms of treatment. However, when the availability of these medications is restricted you must revert to prevention. If you are unaware of the cause of the asthma attacks, start taking notes of everything you did prior to each episode. After several attacks, you may determine what sets them into motion so that you can avoid that action in the future.

ALLERGIC REACTIONS

Allergic reactions occur when the body's immune system is overly sensitive to specific items or groups of items. When at all possible, avoid eating, injecting, touching or breathing in anything you think may cause an allergic reaction. The symptoms can range from itching, rashes, hives, or lumpy patches. Symptoms also include itching and/or burning eyes and a runny nose. Irritation of the throat, difficulty breathing, or even asthma-like symptoms can be a sign of an allergic reaction. Allergic reactions can be very serious and should be identified in the group as part of the planning process. Keep antihistamines on hand for treatment of mild allergies.

Severe allergic reactions can cause anaphylaxis. Having an epinephrine injector on hand is very helpful for the treatment of anaphylaxis. These injectors typically have an 18-month shelf life, but studies have shown that they can still be effective for several years past their expiration date.

BITES

Bites should be treated as open wounds. However, spend more time irrigating the wound. For non-venomous bites, irrigate the wound extremely well with saline or disinfected water. Animal bites are prone to infection. Due to the increased number of loose, hungry dogs and cats during a grid-down situation, animal bites will become more frequent.

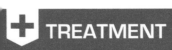

TREATMENT

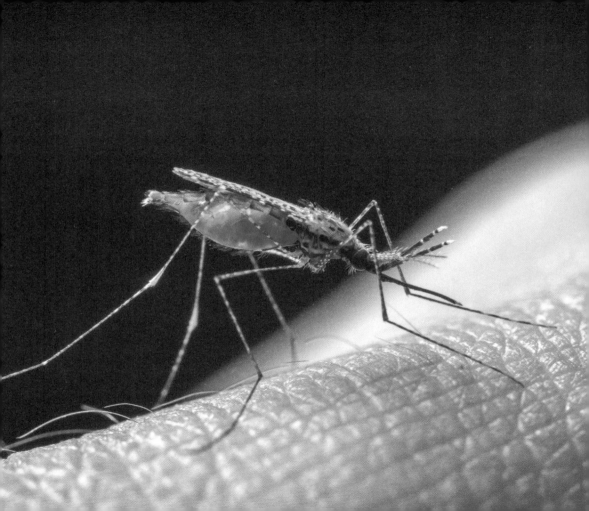

When addressing a venomous bite, immediately clean the area. Not all victims will be injected with venom. Most victims injected with venom report a tingling or metallic taste in the mouth. This symptom typically occurs within minutes, whereas swelling and pain may take up to an hour to occur. Bruising and coloration of the skin will typically occur within several hours and progressively get worse. Immobilize the wounded part of the body below the heart. Wrapping the bitten limb with a bandage may help slow the spread of the venom, but make sure it is not too tight. The bandage should start over the bite and progress evenly toward the torso. The bandage should be loose enough to slide a finger underneath. Venomous bites will cause severe discomfort and can be life threatening during a grid-down situation due to the unavailability of anti-venom.

Other animal bites usually come in three forms: tearing, crushing, and punctures. Some physicians recommend not closing the wound

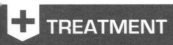

TREATMENT

in an effort to fight infection. However, there are times where closing the wound is necessary to control bleeding. Puncture wounds should not be closed. All bites must be irrigated extensively and allowed to bleed for a moment to help rinse bacteria from the area.

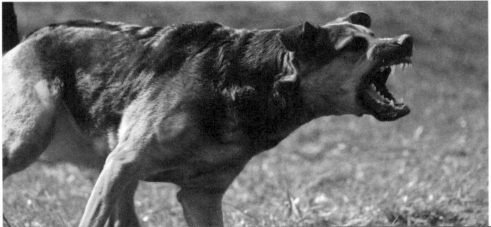

TREATMENT ✚

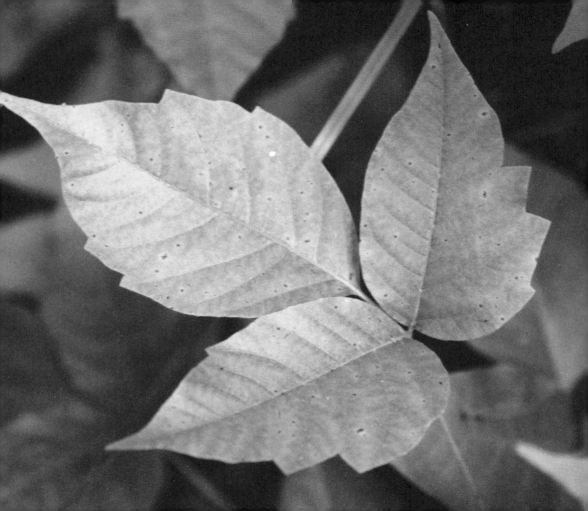

POISON IVY, POISON OAK, AND POISON SUMAC

Poison ivy, poison oak, and poison sumac thrive in many areas of the United States. Each has their own more common areas, but all have similar symptoms and treatment. They all grow leaves in bunches of three. Effects of the toxins can take a few days to become evident. The sticky resin from the leaves can stay active on clothes for extended periods after contact, so handle them with care and launder immediately. The affected area will start as small, severely itchy red bumps, and then become blistered and possibly crusted. The area may streak or become patchy.

Treat the poison affected area by washing throughly with soap and water and then applying topical steroid creams twice daily for 2—3 weeks. Over the counter creams such as Benadryl cream or Calamine lotion can help reduce the itching and may be used as needed. Typically, the rash will clear with three weeks.

TREATMENT ✚

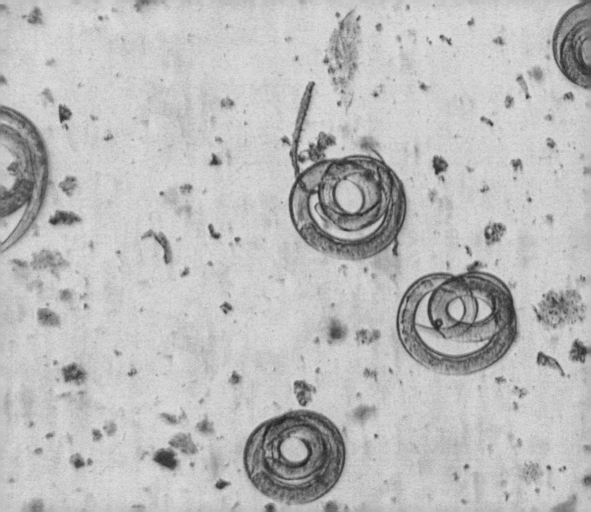

COMMON SICKNESSES

Diarrhea and Dysentery

Main causes of diarrhea are:

- Food poisoning
- Parasites
- Viral or bacterial infections
- Lactose intolerance
- Allergies and food intolerances
- Side effects to medicine
- Eating excess unripe fruit
- Poisonous plants

Loose or watery stool indicates diarrhea, whereas mucus and blood present in fecal matter indicates dysentery. Diarrhea can be serious or mild. The immediate concern is the source of the illness and rehydration of the casualty. Attempt to identify the source of the problem and make sanitary changes to prevent further spread. Check food sources and for exposure to chemicals or plants that may have triggered a reaction. Dysentery is communicable, so quarantine those affected and bleach things and areas they may have contaminated. Diarrhea and dysentery can severely dehydrate and immobilize an entire group. In many cases of diarrhea, no medicine is needed, but careful

TREATMENT +

hydration is required. Dysentery caused by a bacterial infection should be treated with antibiotics, but cases caused by parasites, should be treated with an amoebicidal. In severe cases where the casualty remains dehydrated, utilize an IV to rehydrate. The best prevention is proper nutrition, sanitization, clean water, properly cooked food, and protection of food from flies.

Vomiting

An occasional upset stomach with no apparent cause is common, especially in a survival situation and with children. Your body will go through a dramatic change. Stress, workload, and diet will all dramatically change when the grid goes down. Even after "settling in" you will be exposed to many things that you simply weren't exposed to before. Vomiting can be a sign of many issues—some serious and some minor. Just about any infection or virus can cause vomiting. Gallbladder pain, meningitis, malaria, hepatitis, a urinary infection, and even a migraine can cause vomiting.

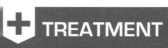

TREATMENT

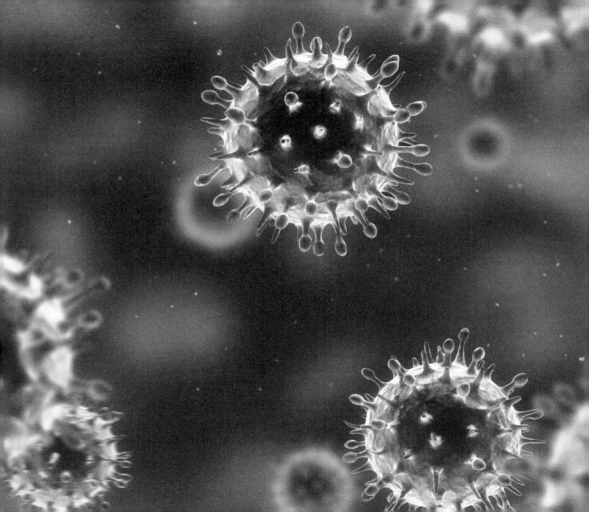

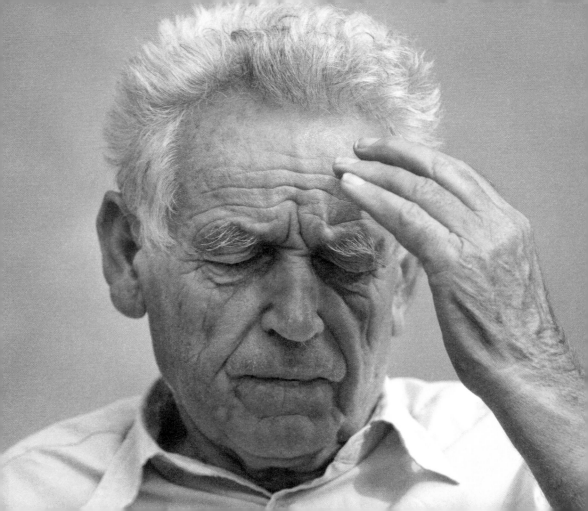

Treatment of vomiting consists of frequent sips on rehydration mix and limiting food intake while vomiting is severe. Common OTC medications include Dramamine, Antivert, or Bonine.

Vomiting can be dangerous if:

- Constant pain persists in the stomach
- Vomiting becomes violent
- Color becomes brown or dark green
- Blood appears in the vomit
- Dehydration increases even with rehydration mix
- Vomit smells like feces

Headaches

Many other conditions can cause headaches that are sometimes referred to as secondary headaches. Dental issues, TMJ, high altitude, heat, sun exposure, or stress may cause these secondary headaches. Headaches are not always a sign of brain issues. Since the brain itself does not have pain receptors, it is likely an irritation of the area around the brain. Sinus irritation or infections often cause headaches. Stay hydrated and protect the head, neck, and eyes from the sun.

Colds & the Flu

Colds and the flu are common viral infections. Antibiotics have no effect on viruses so much needed supplies should not be depleted for colds or flu. Taking antibiotics unnecessarily can even be detrimental, as they eradicate much of the beneficial bacteria in the body along with harmful bacteria. Both cold and flu will usually go away on their own with proper nutrition and hydration. Foods high in Vitamin C may help fight the virus. Do not be misled by the misconception that someone can catch a cold by being cold or wet. Viruses transfer from person to person through mucus, either in the air or on infected surfaces. If possible, separate the infected person from the group or family, especially when sleeping and eating. Cold and flu season is primarily triggered by people remaining indoors and closer to one another than is typical in the summer months.

TREATMENT

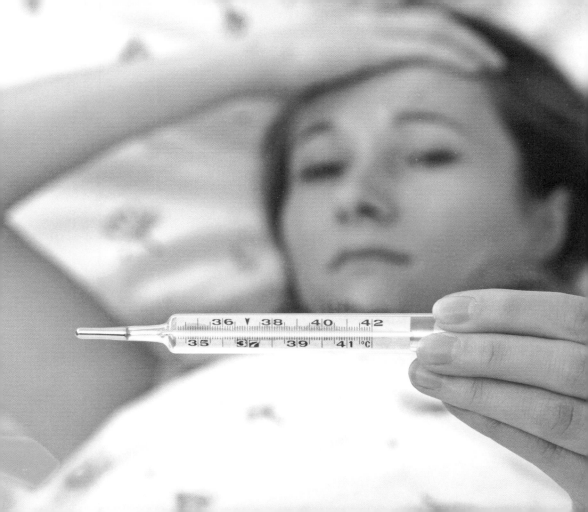

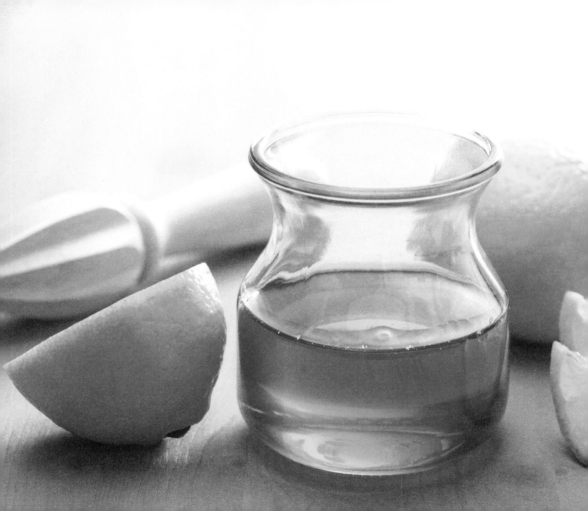

Hay Fever

Hay fever is an allergic reaction to something inhaled from the air. Often this is an issue in the mid to late summer months due to dry grasses and dust in the air. If an antihistamine is available, it can be taken to give temporary relief. Dramamine will sometimes help as well.

Cough

A cough is not a sickness; it is a symptom of a sickness. Coughing is the body's way of cleaning the throat and lungs. If you have a cough, you may not need medicine to stop the coughing. Help loosen the mucus by breathing in hot water vapors several times throughout the day. You can ward off the severity of a cough by taking a mixture that is 1 part honey and 1 part lemon juice. Take one teaspoon every 2-3 hours.

Pneumonia

Pneumonia is an infection in the lungs usually occurring after other respiratory issues. Symptoms of pneumonia are sudden chills and followed by a high fever. Mucus produced by coughing will be yellow, green, reddish or slightly bloody. Casualties will sometimes have chest pain and will appear very weak and pale. Breathing will be rapid and shallow. Grunts and wheezing may be present.

Antibiotics and pain medication are the typical treatments. The person should drink generous amounts of rehydration fluids.

TREATMENT

Swelling of the Feet

Foot swelling can be a major issue as the workload significantly increases for people in a grid-down society. Let's face it; we won't be sitting behind desks anymore. Walking extended distances due to a lack of vehicular transportation and spending extended time standing while holding large amounts of weight will contribute to swollen feet. Keep in mind that if the face or other parts of the body swell as well as the feet, this could be a sign of a more serious illness. Swelling of the feet in small children could be a sign of malnutrition. To treat swelling, you must treat its cause. Reduce or eliminate the use of salt in your diet. When seated, do not sit with your feet below you; prop them up to chest level. When you lie or sleep, keep your feet elevated.

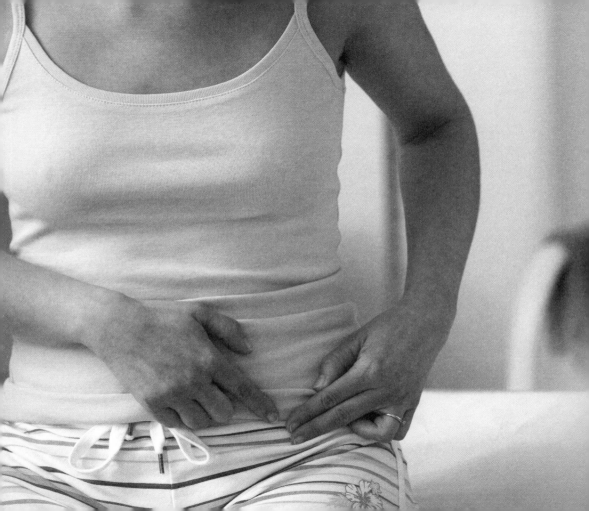

Hernias

Due to the extreme amount of work and the need to move heavy objects in a grid-down situation, an abnormal amount of hernias within your family or group may occur. Prevent this by creating a culture of safety and correcting people when they lift heavy objects incorrectly. They should squat and lift with their legs, NOT bend over and lift with their back. Hernias are tears of the abdomen muscle that allow the intestines to protrude. It should be effective to gently apply pressure to the area, pushing the gut back into the abdomen.

If a hernia becomes large and/or painful, the casualty should lay flat on his back with his legs elevated to a level above his head and gently, but firmly, push it back in. Surgery may be required if the hernia causes vomiting, becomes extremely painful, or the casualty cannot have a bowel movement.

TREATMENT ✚

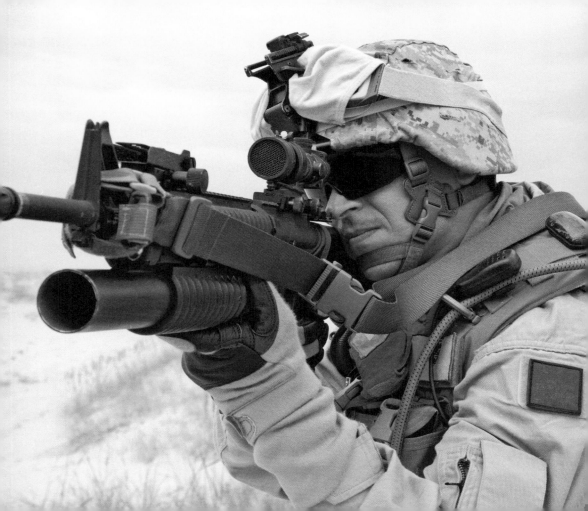

+ BATTLEFIELD AID

In a societal collapse or grid-down scenario, gangs and marauders will likely wreak havoc and chaos around any city regardless of size, by raiding and looting. When people become hungry, they become desperate. You must defend yourself, your family, and your friends in what may become a combat-like scenario. This dramatically increases the risk of battlefield trauma. In this section, we provide some basic knowledge for managing the aid of combat casualties.

Combat casualty care pertains to any situation requiring medical aid within a combat scenario. You and your family defending your structure from hostiles is a good situational example. These hostiles may be well armed or extremely aggressive. Let's say there are only four of you defending a multi-sided structure. Two of you defend the back, and two defend the front. You are 40 feet from your friend across an open driveway and lawn. You see your friend get shot in the leg. Gunfire erupts all around you and your friend. You have the only medical kit. What do you do? Do you help your friend by running over to him and giving him aid, thus putting your wives and children inside the house at risk from the attackers? On the other hand, do you continue the fight and achieve the tactical advantage? This section will help you make those decisions.

The dynamic aspects of grid-down survival will play an extensive role in the type and form of care you provide to yourself and others. Some factors to consider are:

- Gunfire from assaulting force—this may prevent immediate treatment of a wound at the point of injury.

- Equipment availability—many times, you may be limited to what you have on your person.

- Evacuation limits—most likely, evacuation will be impossible. At this point, most hospitals may be completely overrun and non-functioning.

BATTLEFIELD AID

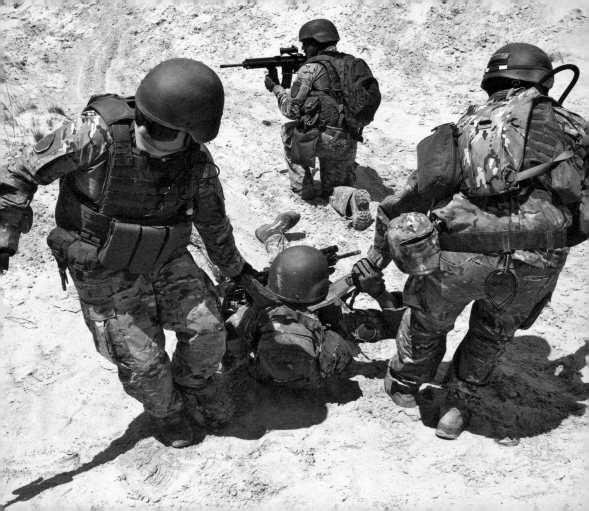

In today's world of moderately trained and well-equipped assaulting forces, the injuries sustained during a grid-down firefight will likely resemble that of the modern battlefield. This requires us to utilize the lessons learned over the last few years of military combat operations.

Modern battlefield wounds that lead to death are most commonly:

- Surgically uncorrectable torso trauma
- Potentially correctable surgical trauma
- Hemorrhage from extremity wounds
- Mutilating blast trauma
- Penetrating traumatic brain injury
- Tension pneumothorax (PTX) (penetrating chest trauma)
- Airway obstruction or injury
- Infection and shock
- Burns

BATTLEFIELD AID

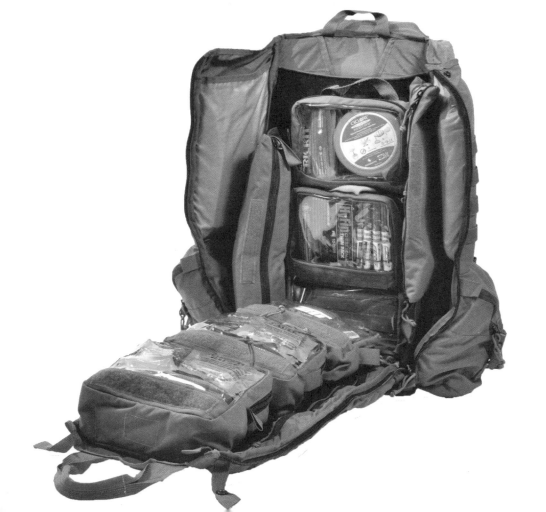

Even with widely available body armor systems, many severe injuries still occur. To manage these injuries, familiarize yourself with the differences between the stages of care and their characteristics.

1st Stage: Care Under Fire
This is care rendered to a person while under enemy fire. The only available equipment is what you carry on your person.

2nd Stage: Tactical Field Care
This is care provided by the group medic once the individuals are no longer under fire. This also refers to the care of a casualty not resulting from enemy fire, but still in a defensive or offensive position or movement.

3rd Stage: Combat Casualty Evacuation
The care provided in movement to an alternate treatment site – possibly to a doctor's house or small community medical facility.

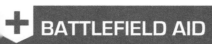

BATTLEFIELD AID

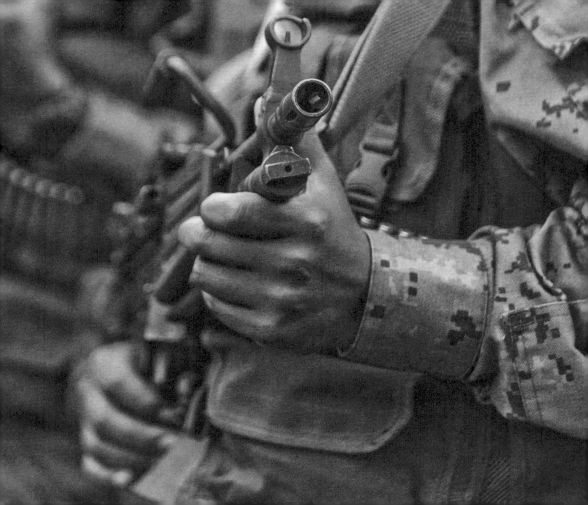

CARE UNDER FIRE

Care under fire is the aid provided to the wounded while receiving hostile fire in close proximity. The risk of additional casualties is extremely high. With such limited personnel, this is typically not a risk worth taking, even to save a life.

The suppression of enemy fire must come prior to attempting any aid. The tactical situation will ultimately dictate the level and timing of care. Do not risk yourself recklessly, as being killed or injured will leave your group's defenses further weakened.

While the group or area is under close enemy fire, the group cannot afford to have a "hero" medic boldly run into hostile fire to save a life or provide a bandage. If the medic becomes injured, who will provide

BATTLEFIELD AID

care for the rest of the group? It will be smarter for the medic to return fire and eliminate further threats. Many times, injuries during a firefight are penetrating extremity injuries. Every member of the group should have a tourniquet and compression bandage. At the very least, the wounded may be able to provide self-aid and return to the fight. Control the bleeding of the non-extremity wounds by the use of pressure dressings. Hemostatic agents and bandages provide a great advantage to stop bleeding.

There may be additional risks associated with attempting the rescue of a casualty.

- Was the casualty a result of an IED (improvised explosive device) designed to draw out medical personnel?

- Was the person a victim of a booby trap?

- Do you have the assets necessary for continued suppressive fire to protect a person rendering aid?

TACTICAL FIELD CARE

This phase of care differs from "care under hostile fire" in that there is more time to provide aid and a decreased hazard of hostile fire. It also applies to the aid of a person who may have been injured by something other than enemy fire. The medical equipment available in this phase still only consists of what the persons have on hand. In many cases, the chance of re-engagement with enemy forces remains high.

The tactical situation will still dictate the management of a casualty. It is more important to accomplish your mission than provide aid. The field medic should always assess his supplies while providing treatment and anticipate re-engagement with enemy forces.

BATTLEFIELD AID

Prior to anyone providing aid, that person must obtain situation awareness, contain the scene, and then assess the casualty.

Treat the casualty by covering these main areas of evaluation:

- **Form a general assessment**—If no one was present to witness the injury, analyze the scene and situation. Take note of the mechanisms of injury. For example, if there is debris everywhere and the victim cannot hear, he may have been the victim of a blast. These notes and observations will help further patient aid.

- **CPR**—If the casualty is unconscious, not breathing, and does not have a pulse by the time you asses him, providing CPR is typically futile. Even if medical help was only minutes away, attempts to resuscitate are rarely successful.

BATTLEFIELD AID ✚

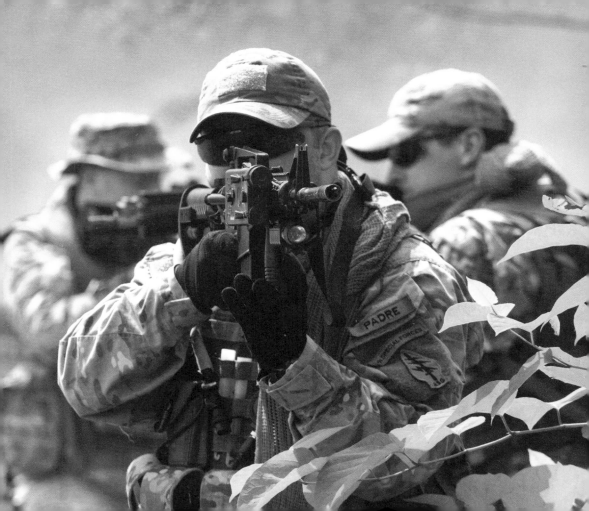

- **Airway Recovery**—Ensure the casualty has no airway restrictions.

- **Breathing**—Remove the casualty's shirt and any armor vest to inspect for puncture, blast, debris, or burns. Note the person's ability to breathe and the equal left/right up and down movement of the chest.

- **Hemorrhage and Circulation**—Assess any tourniquets applied during the care under fire phase. Quickly assess the patient and address any significant bleeding. Re-assess any interventions previously applied.

- **Traumatic Amputations**—Traumatic amputations will not be exclusive to military operations during a grid-down situation. Assess the tourniquet and rinse the wound, thoroughly cleaning any debris. Apply or re-apply dressing and wrap with a bandage.

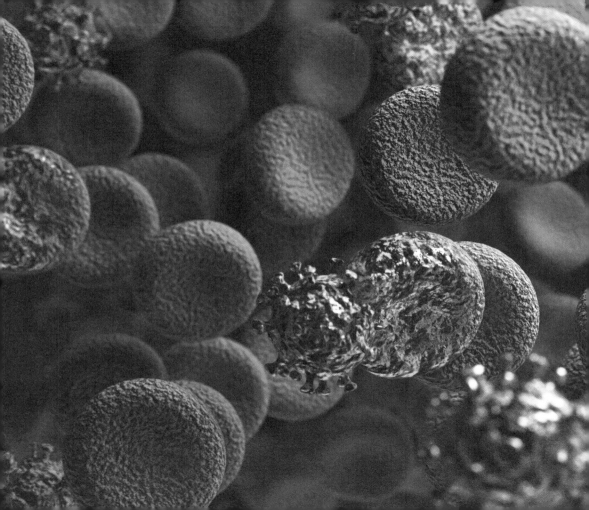

- **Hypothermia**—Regardless of the ambient temperature, most casualties will be susceptible to hypothermia. This is due to heavy blood loss and peripheral vasoconstriction. Utilize anti-hypothermia practices previously discussed.

- **Pain Management**—Everyone deals with pain in his or her own way. Use the medications you have available sparingly. The goal is to reduce the pain and get them back into the fight.

- **Fracture Management**—Examine the wounded by touch, assess the risk of fractures, and splint.

- **Infection Control**—Depending on your level of preparations and stockpile of antibiotics, you may decide the immediate use of antibiotics is best for your group or family. Even on today's battlefield, severe infections remain very common without quickly administering broad-spectrum antibiotics.

BATTLEFIELD AID ✚

While you are assessing the casualty, talk to them. Reassure them that treatment is going well. Tell them what you are going to do. Keep their mind engaged. If they are of sound mind and their conscious state remains stable, have them provide cover. If the conscious state is unstable, remove weapons from them, as they may awaken and mistake you or other friendlies for the enemy.

CASUALTY EVACUATION (CASEVAC) CARE

Evacuation capability in a grid-down situation will be difficult. You will have to modify, improvise, and adjust the normal definition of CASEVAC to fit your capabilities. There will be no Life Flight, no 911 calls, and no ambulance will drive to your front lawn. These services will not be available when the grid goes down. However, the need for evacuation from a firefight area or from the area of a patrol or a recon mission is very likely.

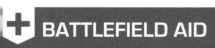 **BATTLEFIELD AID**

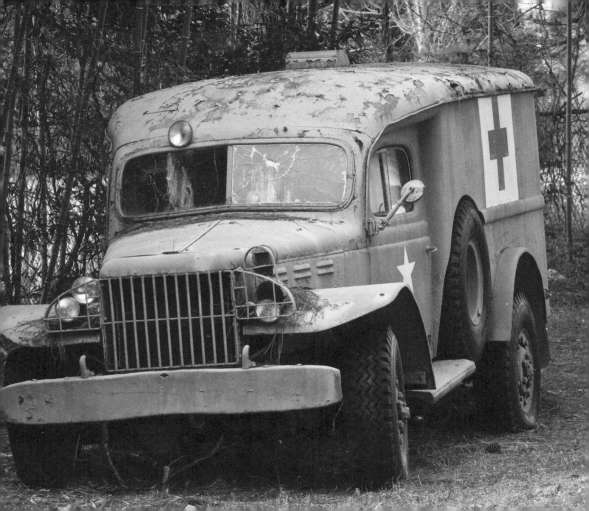

Here is a quick scenario:

People have been approaching your retreat location from a main access road. As a result, your group decides to send a forward team out to observe and provide a warning to the rest of the group if looters approach. The observation site is about one mile north of your retreat location. While setting in to the observation site, the team is attacked. One team member takes a bullet to the chest. He now has a sucking chest wound. The wounded team member retrieves his chest seal, but can't apply it to himself before passing out. After the area is secured, you provide aid to your friend and apply the chest seal after you determine it is necessary. The casualty has short, rapid, and faint breaths. You know he needs a chest decompression needle but the only one the group has is back at the retreat. You and the rest of the team must now evacuate the casualty from the area back to the retreat location. This is when you will begin CASEVAC care.

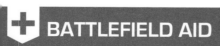

BATTLEFIELD AID

Plan and survey evacuation routes thoroughly. Ensure you have and know your primary, alternate, contingency, and emergency communications plans. Identify possible CASEVAC transfer points. Having a predetermined CASEVAC transfer site will assist in the transfer back to the group.

CASEVAC care is the care provided in en route to the destination. This may require the group's medic to travel with vehicles or a team to gather the casualty. Additional aid and equipment should be available in those vehicles. Re-assess all aspects of the tactical field care.

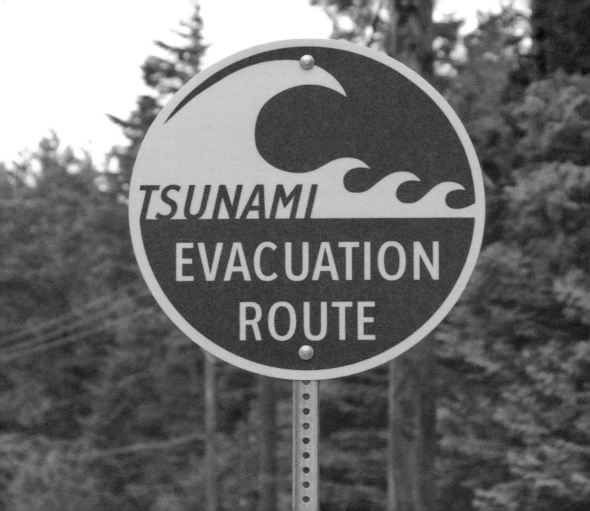

9-LINE CASEVAC

The application of a 9-line CASEVAC is specifically designed for the military and may seem like overkill for civilian use. However, the application and information structure is useful regardless of the societal situation. As any need for a CASEVAC illustrates, having a well-trained group to rely on is the only way to survive in any long-term, grid-down scenario. The following lists the items spoken over a radio to call for a CASEVAC. The location should be given as a grid coordinate, but if this is not available, give the most precise location possible. You may need to use a crossroads or buildings for locations.

The following lists the items spoken over a radio to call for a CASEVAC:

Line 1. Location of the pick-up site. (6-8 digit grid location)

Line 2. Radio frequency, call sign.

Line 3. Number of patients by precedence:
A—Urgent
B—Urgent Surgical
C—Priority
D—Routine
E—Convenience

Line 4. Special equipment required:
A—None
B—Hoist
C—Extraction equipment
D—Ventilator

Line 5. Number of patients by type:
L—Litter (plus number of casualties)
A—Ambulatory (plus number of casualties)

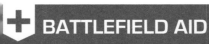

BATTLEFIELD AID

Line 6. Security at pick-up site:

N—No enemy troops in area

P—Possible enemy troops in area (approach with caution)

E—Enemy troops in area (approach with caution)

X—Enemy troops in area (armed escort required)

Line 7. Method of marking pick-up site:

A—Panels (color)

B—Pyrotechnic signal (e.g. red flare)

C—Smoke signal (color)

D—None

E—Other

Line 8. Patient nationality and status:

A—US Military

B—US Civilian

C—Non-US Military

D—Non-US Civilian

E—EPW (enemy prisoner of war)

Line 9. NBC Contamination:

N—Nuclear

B—Biological

C—Chemical

The following is an example of a 9 Line communication:

- "Goose, this is Maverick, over"
- "Maverick, this is Goose. Send your traffic, over"
- "This is Maverick requesting CASEVAC, over"
- "Roger Maverick, send your request, over"
- "Line one, corner of Broadway and 2nd, break"
- "Line two, 462.68750, Maverick, break"
- "Line three, 1B, 3C, 1D, break"
- "Line four, C, break"
- "Line five, 3L, 1A, break"
- "Line six, E, break"
- "Line seven, D, break"
- "Line eight, B, break"
- "Line nine, clear, over"
- "How copy my last, over"
- "Roger Maverick, solid copy, standby for CASEVAC plan, over"
- "Roger, Maverick standing by, over"

✚ BATTLEFIELD AID

+ SUMMARY

The intent of this book is to inform well prepared citizens of basic first aid knowledge that may be necessary in a disaster or grid-down scenario. Although not exhaustive, this guide illustrates some of the most common instances where you may need to employ first aid techniques. Always consult your physician before taking any medications or providing any treatment to yourself or others. Beyond this book, you should continue to gain knowledge and hands-on training to become as proficient as possible. You or your loved ones' lives may depend on this knowledge if the grid goes down.

+ AUTHOR'S BIO

Aaron Iwanciw is a combat veteran with eight years of Marine Corps Infantry experience. He joined the Marine Corps with a passion to fight on the frontlines in defense of our great country. He grew up in the foothills of Middle Tennessee, shooting with his father and attending scout meetings, consistently learning the value of preparedness. As a young boy, Aaron knew he wanted to be a Marine. While many options were available to him, he specifically selected the Marine Corps Infantry. The honest reality of war became personal only a few years later while conducting military force protection operations and countless combat patrols in Iraq. While conducting those duties, he was witness to the consequences of individuals becoming complacent and dependent on government for all they have, making them part of a societal collapse. Observing the effects of chemical changes within desperate and hungry individuals of the populous was life changing. Witnessing frustration turning to aggression and aggression turning to violence changed Aaron's way of thinking forever. Now honorably discharged from the military, Aaron leads his loving wife and two healthy boys in a Christian home in Tennessee. He also leads and conducts the operations of multiple business ventures focused on firearms maintenance, and his consulting firm serves the Department of Defense with combat infantry training in various combat scenarios. It is his pleasure to pull from his life experiences and author this guidebook to help you prepare and address the realities of providing first aid in a grid-down situation.

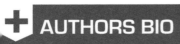